PRAISE FOR *GRATITUDE IGNITION GUIDE*

"Gratitude is simple, but not easy. *Gratitude Ignition Guide* makes an excellent tool for people looking to master how they show up as everyday leaders. Whether you are just starting your gratitude practice, or you're well-versed in it, *Gratitude Ignition Guide* ignites sparks of vitality and joy, and inspires you to embrace gratitude as a character strength, relationship builder, energy generator and a social motivator. By embracing this guide's simple and inspiring messages, you will foster higher levels of thinking, connectivity, and positivity—at home, at work and at play."

—Steve Foran, founder, Gratitude at Work

"Having read Lorraine Widmer-Carson's first book, *An Ecology of Gratitude*, I am pleased to see the release of *Gratitude Ignition Guide*. It provides thoughtful navigation for anyone who is ready to incorporate gratitude into the way they lead. When we go within, relax into and fully experience moments of our lives, gratitude nudges our creative urges, moves us forward and deepens our engagement with life on all levels."

—Karen Close, editor, *Sage-ing With Creative Spirit, Grace and Gratitude, The Journal of Creative Aging*

"Lorraine Widmer-Carson weaves together the power of gratitude and the reflective practice of thoughtful writing as fundamental leadership and personal development tools. In *Gratitude Ignition Guide*, she speaks to the future of everyday leadership, and suggests that leadership is a creative art form. She offers an intelligent, heart-centered, and passionate look at the transformational power of gratitude and personal writing as ways to generate well-being, insight, and growth."

—Lynda Monk, MSW, RSW, CPCC, director of the International Association for Journal Writing

"Thanks to Grassroots Gratitude, I realize the power in meeting with leaders from across Canada who are grappling with questions related to balancing work and life, focusing their energies on what matters, leading in authentic, grounded ways, and many more. I have discovered that an intentional focus on gratitude supports thoughtful decision making, especially as an authentic practice."

—Michelle Schira Hagerman,
associate professor, University of Ottawa

"I've kept a journal since I was a child, and I'm thankful for the many gifts that life has bestowed upon me. It wasn't until I stumbled across Lorraine Widmer-Carson's work that I was able to fully appreciate the power unleashed by combining a conscious gratitude practice with daily journaling. *Gratitude Ignition Guide* is a terrific tool for anyone interested in exploring how introspection and reflection can have a huge impact on creating positive change in all aspects of life. I recommend this guide for team leaders, entrepreneurs, parents, creatives, and anyone who longs to improve the way they show up in the world and, in turn, help make the world a better place."

—Nikki Tate-Stratton, author and
founder of Writers on Fire

"A good journal habit that incorporates gratitude can get me ready for whatever the world is about to deliver. Some days, it can get crazy trying to balance family, projects, and personal time with the needs of my team. Writing longhand and remembering the positives helps me rebound and recalibrate with greater clarity, even when facing significant challenges."

—Steve Ashton, founder and president,
Ashton Construction Services

GRATITUDE
Ignition Guide

NOTES FOR MY LEADERSHIP SELF

LORRAINE WIDMER-CARSON

Copyright © 2023 Lorraine Widmer-Carson

All rights reserved. No portion of this guide may be reproduced, relabelled, or used in any commercial manner whatsoever without the express written permission of the publisher.

For permission contact: lorraine@grassrootsgratitude.ca

Gratitude Ignition Guide: Notes for My Leadership Self

by Lorraine Widmer-Carson
Published by Lorraine Widmer-Carson
Grassroots Gratitude
P.O. Box 1103
Banff, Alberta
Canada

ISBN: 978-1-7777785-2-1

Key Words: Writing Longhand. Journal Practice. Gratitude. Everyday Leadership. Time Management. Decision Making.

Permission is not required for personal or professional use, such as in a coaching or classroom setting.

Printed in Canada

First Edition

Book cover: Lyuba Kirkova, lyubakirkova.com
Book design: Lieve Maas, brightlightgraphics.com
Editor: Dave Jarecki, davejarecki.com

For information about special discounts available for bulk purchases, corporate gifts, philanthropic promotions, fundraising and educational supports, contact the author:
lorraine@grassrootsgratitude.ca

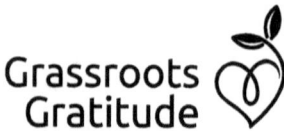

ACKNOWLEDGING THE LAND

I wake up, walk, talk with my family, hear stories from friends, hike and ski within the Treaty 7 territory and Métis Nation of Southern Alberta Region III. I am of English, Scottish and Irish ancestry.

From my earliest days as a child, playing in the hardwood forests of southern Ontario, and paddling lakes lined with Jack pine and birch trees, I have understood that my family and ancestors had immigrated to these places. Our family home in Mt. Pleasant was a rural landscape. Haudenosaunee friends from The Six Nations of the Grand River would often help our parents with chores, then sit with us at the kitchen table, talking as neighbours. I listened to their stories about their families, health concerns, hobbies, and travels. We attended events on reserve that showcased traditions such as "Throwing of the Snow Snake."

My father once asked if a friend's father could translate some English words into their language. I learned the mangled phrase from our friend Roger Porter: "Deka hy-ún ha-dá-saay." This childhood memory dates from a time when my parents were looking to name a piece of property along the Nith River, upstream of its junction with the Grand River, near Mom's hometown of Paris, Ontario. Roger explained that the phrase could really only be spoken. Its meaning is akin to "where the waters meet."

This memory reflects my early understanding of Indigenous relations in Canada. I share it here as part of my continued learning related to conversations on the topic of "Truth and Reconciliation." I invite you to do the same.

With humility and deep respect, I acknowledge that my life has handed me many privileges and gifts beyond what I deserve. I willingly commit and recommit to celebrating gratitude and its transformative power as a character strength that binds us in our tapestry of humanity, as we paddle our individual routes, heading toward those precious places where our waters meet.

CONTENTS

EXECUTIVE SUMMARY   **1**
ABOUT THE *GRATITUDE IGNITION GUIDE*
- Gratitude Is a Force for Change   1
- A Proven Leadership Strength   2
- Writing Your Way Toward Gratitude   5

EVERYDAY LEADERSHIP IS A CREATIVE ART FORM   **9**
- The Great Connector   10
- Finding Gratitude on the Page   11
- This Practice Is Yours Alone   12

YOUR 30-DAY *GRATITUDE IGNITION GUIDE*   **15**

GETTING STARTED   **17**
Day 1: Focus your thoughts   21
Day 2: Right here, right now   22
Day 3: What's your everyday challenge?   23
Day 4: What makes you smile?   24
Day 5: Cycles and seasons   25
Day 6: Your relationship with gratitude   26
Day 7: Benchmarking you   27

DELVING DEEPER   **28**
Day 8: Day off   29
Day 9: After one day off   30
Day 10: Dipping into your memory wells   31
Day 11: Checking your mood   32
Day 12: Checking the mood of your team   33
Day 13: Focus on something small   34
Day 14: Benchmarking you   35

ON EVERYDAY LEADERSHIP — **36**
Day 15: Taking responsibility — 37
Day 16: Quick lists — 38
Day 17: Focusing on positives — 39
Day 18: Acknowledge the negatives — 40
Day 19: Managing time, energy & resources — 41
Day 20: Coaching yourself forward — 42
Day 21: Day off — 43

LEADING WITH STRENGTHS — **44**
Day 22: Benchmarking you — 47
Day 23: No bad days — 48
Day 24: Your best leadership qualities are… — 49
Day 25: What gives you juice? — 50
Day 26: Looking around — 51
Day 27: Take the test — 52
Day 28: Ask a friend or two — 53
Day 29: Pure gratitude — 54
Day 30: Who are you going to thank? — 55
Bonus day: Now to keep going — 56

APPENDIX — **57**
POSTSCRIPT — **60**
CITATIONS — **62**
READING RESOURCES — **64**
ABOUT THE AUTHOR — **65**

EXECUTIVE SUMMARY
ABOUT THE *GRATITUDE IGNITION GUIDE*

Gratitude Ignition Guide invites you to look inside your mind, poke around, and connect the dots that exist between your reality, joys and priorities, in order to find new insight, energy and vitality.

Tapping into gratitude, in the privacy of your thoughts, and without distraction, is a leadership skill that warrants serious consideration. *Gratitude Ignition Guide* helps you do just that, through writing reflectively from the heart. The result is very much like striking a match that can ignite the sparks that connect your mind, hand and heart to your core self and essential truths.

When practiced with intention, gratitude is a life skill that can fuel the fires in your belly, inspiring you to make space for change—personally, socially, and professionally. With deep introspection, you can begin to discern your "core things that matter." By writing about the essential things that bring your life joy and meaning, you risk exposing some soft spots buried deep within. These moments and elements are hinged to your reasons to be grateful and give shape to your larger purpose.

What you'll discover along the way: gratitude can ground you, as well as ignite actions as you give, receive, and recognize the gifts that others bring.

GRATITUDE IS A FORCE FOR CHANGE

Gratitude is more than a greeting card sentiment. It is a compass, a mirror, and a personal calibration lens for viewing life. Gratitude is a complex emotion, a stimulus and response, as well as a character strength. Your reasons to be grateful are rooted in your personal systems of belief, fueled by attitudes and habits of mind that influence your hopes, perspectives, and dreams. It takes intentional effort to understand and unpack your own life stories through a lens of gratitude, but finding your reasons to be grateful can motivate you in the direction of positive change.

Gratitude also demands action. When it fires up, it becomes a generous, life-affirming, relationship-enhancing motivation with pro-social consequences. It inspires positivity, creativity and hope, and broadens your world view.

Gratitude improves relationships at home, in the workplace, on the playing field, and anywhere you go. By giving and accepting gifts in the spirit intended, and by reallocating resources with intentional kindness, grateful leaders can influence the dynamics of every interaction and transaction.

As you shift your relationship to yourself with greater positivity, your relationships with others also shift. As a leader, gratitude positions you to imagine, reach for, and achieve bigger, bolder goals. Ultimately, you flourish in an environment with expanded views of possibilities, connectivity, life purpose, meaning and legacy.

A PROVEN LEADERSHIP STRENGTH

Fostering gratitude is a secret strength in every walk of life, but especially for leaders. There is a bit of irony to this. After all, gratitude is deeply personal, often buried within our souls. Still, gratitude generates maximum benefit when it shines publicly. Writing in a journal is the same: deeply private, intensely personal, but ultimately revealing in your public persona and activities.

Executive Summary About the *Gratitude Ignition Guide*

A positive mindset helps everyone with leadership responsibilities rebound with resiliency when adversity strikes. Standing firm in gratitude puts you back on solid ground. With that said, this isn't just happy-go-lucky, New Age fluff. There's plenty of research-based science related to gratitude. Here are just a few examples that help illustrate this point:

- The character strengths[1] most strongly correlated with well-being, and confirmed by research are Hope, Gratitude, and Love.
- Research[2] also confirms that an effective way to strengthen your gratitude muscles, with the potential to change the shape of your brain,[3] is to write longhand in a journal.[4]
- Keeping a gratitude journal can positively impact your mental health,[5] helping you slow down, focus, process emotions, and organize your thoughts with acuity—something every leader craves.

Author Robert Emmons, authoritative gratitude researcher and founding editor of *The Journal in Positive Psychology*, reports the following in his book, *Gratitude Works!*:[6]

- People are 25% happier if they keep a gratitude journal.
- People who keep gratitude journals sleep 30 minutes longer per evening, and exercise 33% more each week compared to people who do not keep gratitude journals.
- Hypertensives who maintain gratitude journals achieve up to a 10% reduction in systolic blood pressure, and a decrease in dietary fat intake by up to 20%.
- Experiencing gratitude leads to increased feelings of connectedness and altruism, and improves relationships.

Consider the fact that the human brain is made up of a series of electrical impulses and wires managed by our central nervous system. By attempting to shift your thoughts more positively, your brain's neural circuits and hardwires are able to change, thanks to its neuroplasticity. The brain has the ability to reorganize and learn new responses. When you challenge any habitual, quick-firing negativity bias, your grumpy brain can look for and find new, more positive thought patterns.

With intention, time and practice, it is possible to shift your neural circuits and mental wavelengths in the direction of greater positivity, thereby silencing your inner critics, and improving your coping mechanisms. Through the process of writing daily, and seeking gratitude, you may also ignite the following:

- With gratitude, you discover more reasons to be positive and engaging, and you enjoy greater life-satisfaction.
- Grateful people are less materialistic, and more grounded in their happiness. Studies show that materialistic people are less happy.[7] Your need for "retail therapy" or "self-medications" may dwindle.
- Gratitude is an antidote to anxiety, worry, loneliness, and depression. You may achieve a higher mental health baseline. Gratitude is a natural anti-depressant with no known negative side effects.
- With a reduction in stress levels, your heart becomes healthier, and your cortisol levels drop.
- In a society that may overvalue privacy, gratitude offers a warming glow, illuminating your self-worth in the context of your social group.
- Gratitude can also help you manage your time, as in: time to be alone; time for being with others; time for working, playing and talking to new people; time to intentionally choose and manage your time for personal reasons.
- Your emotional pendulum may swing in the direction of "good enough." There is a decision-making tool that

Executive Summary About the *Gratitude Ignition Guide*

mixes the words "satisfy and suffice." Constantly seeking perfection is often a route to frustration, disappointment, resentment, and burnout. If you find it difficult to realize complete satisfaction, perhaps you can aspire to becoming "satisficed."
- You may begin to recognize privileges and gifts of benevolence that you hadn't noticed before.
- More smiles may come your way. Your body will be flushing with higher levels of dopamine, serotonin, and oxytocin, the feel-good hormones. You will smile more easily, and interactions with others will become friendlier.
- With an improved understanding of yourself and others, your emotional intelligence will increase. You may become more empathetic, co-operative, and self-compassionate, and your relationships will flourish.

WRITING YOUR WAY TOWARD GRATITUDE

Writing longhand is a full-body experience. At times, it is physical, emotional, spiritual, and intellectual. It is a process that links your head, hand, and heart to the past, present, and future.

When approached on a regular basis, and writing about "your things that matter," you find more reasons to be grateful. In the process, you deepen your joys and lighten your burdens.

This guide urges you to write longhand, with a paper and pen, for at least 11 minutes a day. Spend your first minute getting ready, then give yourself at least 10 minutes to write. From the comfort of a private, calm, well-lit desk (preferably first thing in the morning), you can stave off the impulse of electronic devices, and let your journal be a vessel for collecting thoughts and emotions. From there, you can mix them in the fertile soil of your memories, dreams, stories, imagination, beliefs and goals.

The goal: To dedicate and intentionally make time to focus your attention, enjoying the practice of writing longhand.

The outcome: By focusing on what's happening in your life (the good and bad) you will discover many layers to your beliefs, thoughts, attitudes, strengths, and emotions. You will start to see some inconsistencies, and may discover some untruths. As you gain greater self-awareness, you will be recalibrating, re-wiring, and revitalizing your personal leadership style.

It's been a pleasure creating this *Gratitude Ignition Guide* in support of your learning and development journey. Once you decide this pursuit is worth your time, talent, and attention, be sure to celebrate and tell others about your personal revelations. As the famous Gertrude Stein saying goes, "Silent gratitude isn't much use to anyone."

Lorraine Widmer-Carson

Lorraine

September 15, 2023

"Between stimulus and response there is a space. In that space is our power to choose our response. In our response lies our growth and our freedom."

—Viktor Frankl

EVERYDAY LEADERSHIP IS A CREATIVE ART FORM

A thoughtful, reflective leadership style grounded in gratitude brings insight, self-awareness, and honesty—whether times are good or otherwise. Even though there is no one set of rules when it comes to leadership, we can all agree that communities thrive when we care about the quality of relationships—individual to individual, and organization to organization.

There are many examples of everyday leaders doing wonderful things in the world. They understand the importance of positive flow; they deftly build bridges that connect people, places, policies, and process; they are smart, savvy, self-aware, sentient, and exhibit a strong social conscience.

Such leaders create conditions for deep, evolving, inclusive and urgent conversations. They imagine living together in ways that encourage mutual respect, building trust, and responding sensitively to changing conditions and transitions.

The world is aching for more leaders who understand that life is an ebb and flow, and who possess emotional intelligence that enables them to lead with compassion and empathy. We applaud leaders who recognize their character strengths, and embrace the strengths of others, aware that their decisions are critical to the collective.

At home, in a family, on a team, or just on daily walk-abouts, we need to see ourselves as everyday leaders, influencing and impacting each other.

To paraphrase one of my favourite articles on leadership: everyday leadership occurs when each of us takes intentional, daily action to foster better connection, communication, and community, to share a vision that we can do better together. The challenges we face are significant, and headwinds are strong. The entire team, from CEO down, can and must find new ways to align efforts, and make the world better for future generations.[8]

THE GREAT CONNECTOR

Gratitude connects us to each other, binding us in a myriad of relationships. It occupies a place in our hearts that is very close to love, loss, and grief. With gratitude, we become appreciative of the things we risk losing, or may have already lost. Understanding the power of gratitude in your life is likely to be transformative and energizing, full of potential energy, even in times of pain.

In her book, *Finding the Mother Tree*,[9] Suzanne Simard explains her understanding of natural cycles at work in the old-growth forest. Her ground-breaking research confirms that mycorrhizal fungi play a vital role in the nutrient exchange processes during growth, decline, decay, and reciprocity between living systems above and below ground.

The sub-soil transference of carbon, nitrogen, amino acids, and sugars, recycling nutrients between individuals, as well as between species, gives the forest a kind of intelligence. Simard draws comparisons to our human systems of social/psycho/neuro/biological function. Like the forest, we thrive when our natural processes are functioning well, even in the aftermath of disruption, extraction, or interference.

I am also reminded of the book *Authentic Happiness*, by Dr. Martin Seligman. In it, Dr. Seligman describes the student assignment that includes writing a thank-you letter, then speaking the thank-you aloud in front of a class. The person being thanked is in attendance. About this gratitude night, Seligman writes, "the givers, the receivers, the observers all cried. When starting to cry, I didn't know why I was crying. Crying in any class is extraordinary, and when everyone is crying, something has happened that touches the great rhizome underneath all humanity."[10]

FINDING GRATITUDE ON THE PAGE

If you are new to writing in a journal, a good way to motivate yourself and stick with the habit is to consider it a part of your identity. If you want to show up and identify as a confident, self-aware, and socially conscious person who lives in alignment with your core values, then keeping a journal is an excellent habit to hone.

As you invest more time and energy toward building a writing practice, your inside voices gain confidence, clarity, and courage. There are no known harmful side effects to being grateful, assuming you practice it with honesty, humility, and integrity. By allowing your voices of self-sabotage and negativity to take a well-deserved break, you will be learning to play to your strengths, reducing your focus on mistakes or weaknesses.

Writing in a journal is a splendid way to spark a deeper sense of curiosity, imagination, awe, creativity—and yes, gratitude. At any moment, feel free to pen the words: "I wonder, I wonder…" Then, meander along some newly inspired paths of speculative fiction, in the privacy of your pages.

Through the habit of writing longhand, and keeping a running tally of your gifts, joys, challenges, and anxieties, you can find new energy to stand tall. But fair warning: writing takes time, and this habit requires commitment, focus and self-discipline. A deeply reflective writing practice may also bring you closer to tender places and vulnerable spots buried deep in your subconscious. Be patient. Be gentle with yourself. Being grateful demands courage as you keep going.

THIS PRACTICE IS YOURS ALONE

The act of writing is part imagination, part factual, and completely fantastical, delivering its own type of magic. Consider adopting an identity that says, "I am an everyday leader who enjoys the experience of writing." Stay curious. Keep showing up at the page.

There is no right way to do anything that follows. Your imagination is your best fire starter. Finding the thoughts and ideas that are ready to burn is like stacking kindling. The prompts in this guide are encouragements. The embers that your pen stirs up are yours to manage, to use as fuel to keep going, or to dampen if they cause pain.

There is no pressure, but make a commitment to pay attention, and stay aware of your mood, energy, and physical shifts. Choose your words and thoughts carefully. Sometimes, you may need to find a better word that expresses your idea more creatively, more accurately. The goal: to seek greater clarity in word, thought, and action.

Avoid being stuck in a looping state of reactivity, anxiety, or confusion. That said, there may be moments of writing when you find yourself unpacking challenges. Emotions will become volatile, while facts prove elusive. Such is life. Writing exposes our inconsistencies and false assumptions!

Stay with the process, even if it takes longer to understand where you want your writing to go. You may need to do more research, dig deeper, or reframe your thoughts around new questions. Give yourself permission to fan or douse ideas; pause at any moment if you need to recalibrate in the changing winds of circumstance or understanding.

As you start your journal writing practice, you may notice some shifts around day 14. They say it takes at least 30 uncomfortable days to form a new habit. Other theorists suggest that it takes at least 21 days to start forming a habit, and an additional 90 days for the habit to become sustainable.

No matter your view or starting point, this guide will help you gain a new appreciation for the art of writing longhand—one that brings you to a threshold of grateful insight and inspiration. Commit to a goal of writing every day for at least 14 days, then see what happens. Can you continue for another week after that? That gets you to 21 days. From there, can you make it all the way to 30?

With gentle encouragement and great optimism, I hope you enjoy the process.

"The purpose of life is not to be happy. It is to be useful, to be honorable, to be compassionate, to have it make some difference that you have lived and lived well."

—Ralph Waldo Emerson

YOUR 30-DAY GRATITUDE IGNITION GUIDE

"The palest ink is better than the best memory."

—Chinese proverb

GETTING STARTED

With a deeper understanding of mutual relatedness, everyday leaders can help each one of us stand taller, and bring out the best in one another. Please don't take my word for it. You must prove this for yourself.

Your 30 days of writing prompts follow. Use the space provided as an invitation to begin each day's session. Be mindful of moments when you're called to pivot, even if only as a thought exercise.

Some final notes before you begin:

- Start each writing session with a positive mindset, and a personal declaration that this is your private practice. Thoughts are not facts. Let emotions flow.
- Consider writing any private thoughts that need more time and attention in a separate journal. Go so far as to label a separate journal "Confidential" if that helps remove the risk of someone else reading it.
- You may want to have a conversation with your partner or house-mates, framing the habit as a personal growth opportunity.
- Be patient with yourself. Find the place and time of day that works best for you.
- Commit to showing up at the page every day. If you are writing in the morning, you may start by revelling in your private thoughts, recording dreams or sleepy ideas. Soon you will get past your dream-state. As your thinking becomes more organized, use the prompts to prepare for the day ahead, with a positive mindset. Even on the days that

Gratitude Ignition Guide

- you have zero minutes, pull out this guide and write the date, time, and one tiny thing.
- These prompts will fuel one element of your daily ritual. Another part of your writing practice might delve into a deeper, more introspective brain space. For thoughts that cause a pivot, cultivate your practice further by writing fearlessly and honestly, nudging closer to greater clarity, calm, and self-confidence.
- When putting pen to paper, you may notice that your self-limiting beliefs and negativity biases are the first to arrive. This is normal. We are all hardwired with negatives. There may even be a chorus of voices ringing in the hallways of your head, sabotaging good ideas. With time and effort, positives will rise.
- Set your intentions by calming any voices of negativity and skepticism. Listen for the small voice of innocence that whispers, "Okay, this is just me talking with a pen in hand, a fire in my belly, a willingness to try, and permission to dream."
- As your practice grows, get more curious. Keep refining and customizing your journal practice in a way that invites new inspiration and fresh ideas.
- This exercise demands that you slow yourself down, unplug from the world and place a "Do Not Disturb" sign on the door to your office. It asks you to write notes to yourself, by yourself, with free rein to exaggerate the truth, imagine with creativity, and assume full permission to relax.
- Consider this a timed workout: no music, no mirrors, and no one else is in the gym. You are alone with your thoughts.
- Find a good work surface, a pen, this book, and maybe another journal to keep nearby. Keep looking for your sense of joy, humour and playfulness, even on dark days.

- Take a few cleansing breaths. Soften your gaze. Remove your blinders. Let go of your filtered thoughts. Enjoy moments of creativity and spontaneity as they come. The harness of duty and obligation to others can wait. This is about you.
- Every day, look for glimmers of hope and tiny moments of joy. When someone thanks you or acts in a way that is considerate and tender, ask yourself: Is that an expression of gratitude? For example: a bouquet of flowers or a text that simply says "Thinking of you."

DAY 1: FOCUS YOUR THOUGHTS

Start by thinking about what is going well in your life, at work, personally, professionally…wherever the good is coming from. Begin with the phrase, "Five things for which I am most grateful." Close by noting the following: "One thing I really want to do today."

....
....
....
....
....
....
....
....
....
....
....
....
....

Getting something down on paper is a great start. If you have time to keep writing, continue today's session by adding some "notes to self" in the form of bullet lists, word clouds, mind maps, or doodles in your other journal.

DAY 2: RIGHT HERE, RIGHT NOW

What's top of mind right now? People? Relationships? Hobbies? Schedules? What are you most excited about today? What will it mean to get this done?

....

....

....

....

....

....

....

....

....

....

....

....

What else is piquing your curiosity? Fire up your imagination by remembering something that's in your coat pocket, or waiting by the door. Then keep writing, using some good words. From there, challenge yourself to find even better words.

DAY 3: WHAT'S YOUR EVERYDAY CHALLENGE?

Our routines, rituals, and habits help us manage our time, energy and resources. What's your best strength when facing one of your usual challenges?

....
....
....
....
....
....
....
....
....
....
....
....
....
....

Are you dreading something that's pending? Do you need to make a final decision on something? Can you find the words to express something hiding in the shadows?

DAY 4: WHAT MAKES YOU SMILE?

"Today I am smiling because…" My playful expression for this exercise is "tut comms," an acronym for "turning up the corners of my mouth." What things make you smile? How many "tut comms" can you list in a hurry?

_____

_____

_____

_____

_____

_____

_____

_____

_____

_____

_____

_____

If you're stuck, here's another playful exercise. Put your pen between your teeth. Without letting your lips touch the pen, go look in the mirror. See? You're smiling! What else is in there? "I always smile when…"

DAY 5: CYCLES AND SEASONS

Write today's date. Scan through your nearest calendar. Check out last month, this month, and the next. By quickly glancing through the recent past, present, and future, consider how your leadership duties have varied in the last 60 days. "When I look back, I am delighted to note…" "When I look ahead, I am excited to think…" How does this translate over the course of a full year?

....

....

....

....

....

....

....

....

....

....

....

....

Are your activities as a leader gearing up? Winding down? Stuck in neutral? Are you training for something in the future? Are you in a season of growth or decline? Is your team expanding? Shrinking? What else?

DAY 6: YOUR RELATIONSHIP WITH GRATITUDE

Start some lists. Feel free to embellish in the days to come:

- Gifts I bring to the table…these are my strengths.
- Ways I like to shine…these are my joys.
- How I like to celebrate team or group wins…these are the ways I appreciate others.
- Things that make me happy…these are my simple pleasures.

Write the words: "I remember this unexpectedly beautiful thing that happened when…" Keep writing about that unexpectedly beautiful thing.

DAY 7: BENCHMARKING YOU

You're 7 days into your practice. Well done. It's time to score yourself on the following criteria:

Energy: 0 = Depleted, exhausted. 10 = Over the top.
Relaxation: 0 = I can't relax. My brain is like a squirrel on steroids. 10 = I am savouring everything.
Happiness: 0 = I am so low, my chin is touching the ground. 10 = Look out world, I am taking charge.

....
....
....
....
....
....
....
....
....
....
....
....
....

Did anything shift this week? Has this journal writing practice altered your perspective? How so? Positively? Negatively? Lean into this thought, then write on.

DELVING DEEPER

Self-leadership becomes everday leadership. By writing in a journal, you are growing your sense of self-awareness and self-acceptance. When you understand your personal priorities, motivations, and reasons for doing what you do, you become aligned with knowing what you love. You also begin to see how you might be getting in your own way (procrastination, avoidance, self-sabotage, etc.).

When we write in a journal, we often bump into memories, old beliefs, hard-wired habits, and tired clichés. In the days to come, challenge yourself to find new ways to say the same old thing. For instance, what's one of your go-to clichés? Are you a "sure thing" person? Do you tend to answer questions with "no problem"? Do you find yourself saying "can't complain" when people ask how your day is going?

You might be doing something similar in your writing practice. As you write, ask yourself: "Do I really believe what I just wrote? Is there another way to write it?" Can you find a better word? A kinder thought? A gentler way of being with yourself?

Here's something else to consider: We often misremember dates, events, faces and so on. Our memories are actually quite shoddy. Don't be surprised if your memory of an event differs from a friend's memory of the same moment. Relax and accept…such is life!

You can still be the hero of your own story. Your memory is yours to savour and store in a sacred place. You don't need to change the memory if it's an honest and valid self-reflection. With that said, the same holds true for the other person.

DAY 8: DAY OFF

Today is a well-earned day off from writing. Instead, I offer a challenge: Stay as unplugged from your devices as possible. Obviously, if it's a work day, you'll be checking email, going to meetings, and even conversing with colleagues or clients via any number of apps. Track how much time you spend on technology. Notice where you lose yourself. How can you gain some of this time back, whether today or in the future?

If you really want to write something, don't hold back. Make it creative. Write down the lyrics of a song or a poem that's looping in your head. Describe a piece of art. Make note of a poster or bumper sticker that recently caught your attention.

DAY 9: AFTER ONE DAY OFF

How did it feel to not write yesterday (assuming you didn't)? What did you do during your unplugged time? Did you win any time back? Did you go outside? Read a book? Meditate? Talk to someone? Savour something special?

....
....
....
....
....
....
....
....
....
....
....
....

After 9 days, what's your best time of day to write? How long do you write? What coaching tips can you give yourself in order to keep showing up at the page?

DAY 10: DIPPING INTO YOUR MEMORY WELLS

Think of a time when you felt large and in charge as a leader. When you show up as your best self, what are you doing? What are your feelings? Calm? Confident? Slightly nervous? Describe one single moment that illustrates the way you want others to see you. Savour this moment today.

....
....
....
....
....
....
....
....
....
....
....
....
....

Did someone share this moment with you? For fun, ask them to recount their version of the same story. Here's a simple way to get started: "What do you remember about…?" Listen intently. Let them tell their version of the story. Stay open-minded and curious.

DAY 11: CHECKING YOUR MOOD

How are you feeling? Happy? Sad? Calm? Stressed? All of the above? Are you feeling positive and optimistic? Negative and cranky? There's no right or wrong way to feel, especially since our emotions are complex and multi-coloured. Still, it is worth noting that negative emotions are usually related to something past or future. Right here, right now, in this very moment, we can usually find positivity. Some prompts to get going:

- I would really like to start by saying that…
- Which means I am feeling…
- I am happy that…
- My focus today will be…

....

....

....

....

....

....

....

Whenever you need to narrow your focus quickly and positively, use this prompt:

- Five things I am seeing
- Four things I am feeling
- Three things I am hearing
- Two things I am smelling
- One thing I am savouring, which is like saying, "I am grateful for…"

DAY 12: CHECKING THE MOOD OF YOUR TEAM

When you work alongside others, their moods, feelings and concerns will impact you. Thinking about your team, what is the general mood? Happy? Sad? Calm? Stressed? Why? Does it relate to the past? Present? Future?

....
....
....
....
....
....
....
....
....
....
....
....
....

After considering your team as a group, focus on one or two individuals. Who is the most positive and optimistic person you interact with? Who is the adorable curmudgeon? How do the emotional swings of others impact you? Remember to keep private anything that someone else might find hurtful. If you haven't used your other journal yet, today is a good day to open it.

DAY 13: FOCUS ON SOMETHING SMALL

Narrow your sights to something very simple and small. Tighten your focus to right here, right now. Describe something on your desk, in your drawer, or even a mark on your hand. Use as many descriptive details as possible: colour, shape, texture, size, etc. Be specific. Enjoy using simple words.

....

....

....

....

....

....

....

....

....

....

....

....

....

....

Now, go big by broadening your focus. Describe the scene out the window or beyond your desk. Be as accurate and descriptive as possible, using bigger words if they arise.

DAY 14: BENCHMARKING YOU

You're 14 days into your practice. Great work. It's time to score yourself again, using the same criteria as on Day 7:

Energy: 0 = Depleted, exhausted. 10 = Over the top.
Relaxation: 0 = I can't relax. My brain is like a squirrel on steroids. 10 = I am savouring everything.
Happiness: 0 = I am so low, my chin is touching the ground. 10 = Look out world, I am taking charge.

Did anything shift this week? Has this journal writing practice altered your perspective in any way? Write on.

ON EVERYDAY LEADERSHIP

Implicit in the idea of leading others is the demand to know yourself. Sadly, humans are notoriously bad at knowing what is good for us. That's according to the world's longest scientific study of happiness.

To borrow a quote from the book, *The Good Life*, "Life, even when it's good, is not easy. There is simply no way to make life perfect. Why? Because a good life is forged from precisely the things that make it hard."[11]

This guide explores the power of writing in a journal as an essential tool. As you go deeper, you continue to distinguish yourself as an open-minded, curious person who possesses a growth mindset. You are willing to reflect on the many factors at play in your life, and in the lives of others.

Sadly, there is no "happy button" to press that will help you stay in your happy place. To flourish, you must work with the negatives as well. Learning from mistakes and navigating adversity are just two of the ways in which you can grow and learn.

As you do your work in the world, you will continue to find greater meaning and purpose by experiencing positives and negatives. As the saying goes, "No rain, no rainbows."

DAY 15: TAKING RESPONSIBILITY

Write about your kind of everyday leadership. Start by writing yourself some leadership coaching notes. Find words for coaching yourself, and words to use when coaching others.

....
....
....
....
....
....
....
....
....
....
....
....
....

Think of a time when you positively impacted others. What did you do? Write your own hero story, with you in the lead role.

DAY 16: QUICK LISTS

Note your mood before you start today. What is the reason? What is the season? Make a list of at least five things you are savouring right now. Gadgets? Sunsets? Food? New activities? What's giving you juice, and getting you energized?

....

....

....

....

....

....

....

....

....

....

....

....

....

....

Note your mood as you put your pen away and think about getting more of those savoury feelings.

DAY 17: FOCUSING ON POSITIVES

Make a list with three positives and one negative currently affecting your leadership duties. In what ways are you flourishing? Are your tides rising and coming in? Or are you in a phase of the moon where the tides are going out? Metaphorically speaking, what is the weather forecast? How are you getting ready?

....

....

....

....

....

....

....

....

....

....

....

....

Go back to Day 4 and reflect on the things that turned up the corners of your mouth. What is bringing a smile to your face today?

DAY 18: ACKNOWLEDGE THE NEGATIVES

Negatives abound for everyone. How are you balancing the good with the bad? With the ugly? What is your ratio of good to bad things? Write a quick list of things going well, then another for the things going sideways. Note: It is recommended to aim for a Positivity Ratio of at least three heartfelt positive emotions that uplift you, for every gut-wrenching negative experience.[12]

....

....

....

....

....

....

....

....

....

....

....

A toxic culture results when people are overly competitive, self-centred, and display judgemental or perfectionist tendencies. A toxic workplace breeds inefficiency, cynicism, irresponsibility, and skepticism. What is your advice for everyday leaders who want to infuse teams with greater productivity, positivity, and efficiency?

DAY 19: MANAGING TIME, ENERGY & RESOURCES

What's on your to-do list today? Use your journal to make some solid decisions related to managing your time, energy, and resources, whether human, social, or financial. Try using the 4-D method: Do, Delete, Delegate, or Delay.

....
....
....
....
....
....
....
....
....
....
....
....

Who do you need to communicate with about your 4-D decision? Deciding to delete or delay are still decisions that have consequences. Deciding to delegate means you need to ask someone to pick up the slack for you.

DAY 20: COACHING YOURSELF FORWARD

What are today's burning issues? What tools are helpful as you unpack the issues and get to the good stuff? Meditation? Exercise? Nature? Talking to a trusted colleague? Taking a nap? A good morning routine is like having a good breakfast.

....

....

....

....

....

....

....

....

....

....

....

....

....

When writing about deeper issues, consider moving your pen to your "confidential" notebook. Staying with your writing, and reframing when necessary, can help you get to the bottom of what's on your mind. However, it takes discipline, practice and persistence. Keep seeking the positives, and be patient with yourself.

DAY 21: DAY OFF

Today is a second well-earned day off from writing (remember Day 8?). Here's the same challenge as last time: Stay as unplugged as possible. Pay attention to your daydreams and emotions as they come and go. Enjoy your own company.

While you're not writing (and not scrolling), go for a stroll. Make a plan to connect with a friend. Reach out to someone you want to share time with, or to whom you wish to give a gift of appreciation. Notice how doing something kind for others makes you feel.

LEADING WITH STRENGTHS

Leadership is a creative art form, and a character strength. Leadership is also about relationships. When done well, it is an expression of who you really are—the authentic you.

To lead with strength and clarity, you must recognize your strengths. You must also realize that you have some weaknesses.

When working with others, you can bring your strong suits, and acknowledge that other people bring different sets of tools and talents. As you work, interact, and lead together, you build your individual and collective levels of resiliency, flexibility, and co-creativity.

Thinking about character strengths[13] can increase a group's understanding of diversity, equity, acceptance, inclusion, humility, and tolerance, framed through a lens of gratitude.

As you're discovering through this process, gratitude is a complex psycho-social-spiritual-physical response that has various benefits. It's also a habit that takes practice, along with an open mind. Let's keep building it.

Our character strengths are the things that make us human, and the universal qualities that define us. They include things like Kindness, Gratitude, Love of Learning, and the Appreciation of Beauty and Excellence. You'll find a full list of 24 strengths in the Appendix.

Among the strengths that have been identified as game changers in the context of well-being and flourishing are:

- Hope & Optimism
- Gratitude
- Curiosity
- Social Intelligence
- Self-control (Self-regulation)
- Perseverance (Grit)
- Enthusiasm (Zest)

We each have strengths, as well as biases. We are full of contradictions, paradoxes, and inconsistencies. There is a lot sloshing around in our heads: memories, voices, ideas, and belief systems meshed in with cultural bias. We need to stay gentle with ourselves, and remain tolerant of others as our neurons fire and hormones flush through.

With time and practice, you can learn to understand yourself better, get closer to defining your true self, and discover what helps you cultivate a mindset that is happy, calm, content, and confident.

Your core self is that which defines your essence. This is an essential piece to nurture and cultivate as you show up in your leadership role. In the end, self-leadership leads to stronger leadership. Self-awareness helps you pause and take a moment to articulate clearly, and find a better word even when tensions run high.

Gratitude Ignition Guide

During the coming week, recognize when various emotional responses are rising. Look at this list of eight C's[14] and notice what you are doing when you feel any of these (in combination, or on their own).

- Calm
- Clear
- Curious
- Connected
- Confident
- Compassionate
- Creative
- Courageous

DAY 22: BENCHMARKING YOU

It's time to score yourself again, using the same criteria as Days 7 and 14:

Energy: 0 = Depleted, exhausted. 10 = Over the top.
Relaxation: 0 = I can't relax. My brain is like a squirrel on steroids. 10 = I am savouring everything.
Happiness: 0 = I am so low, my chin is touching the ground. 10 = Look out world, I am taking charge.

How has your journal writing practice contributed to your score? Look back to Days 7 and 14. How have your numbers changed? In what ways? Now, let's write another list, labeled: "Reasons I want to keep my writing habits..."

DAY 23: NO BAD DAYS

Think about the seas you are in right now. Describe your watercraft. Are you floating, paddling, passenger, or captain? From paddle board to life raft, consider your C's (from the earlier "C list"). Play with the following idea: "My eight C's and I may encounter some stormy seas today. My best strengths for keeping my boat afloat are..."

....

....

....

....

....

....

....

....

....

....

....

....

Which one of the eight C's is easiest for you to experience? Which is the most difficult? Which C presents the greatest opportunity for your personal growth and development? Which C remains most elusive for you to feel?

DAY 24: YOUR BEST LEADERSHIP QUALITIES ARE...

Refer to the list of 24 Character Strengths[15] summarized in the Appendix. Do a self-analysis, and select your top five strengths. Write them here.

....
....
....
....
....
....
....
....
....
....
....
....

Who has influenced your understanding of gratitude? Who is the most grateful person you know? As a leader, how do you like to demonstrate appreciation for the efforts of others? How often? Anything else?

DAY 25: WHAT GIVES YOU JUICE?

Stepping up with self-confidence, clarity, courage, and compassionate-awareness is easier when you play to your strengths, in alignment with your true self. Describe the strengths you bring to the table all day, every day.

....
....
....
....
....
....
....
....
....
....
....
....

Negative energy is another kind of juice. How often do you use swear words? At whom or what are you usually swearing? Do you admonish others in the same voice that you admonish yourself? What are some better words to use when you need to express your bleeps and expletives?

DAY 26: LOOKING AROUND

Returning to the list of 24 Character Strengths, name the people in your world who display strengths you admire and aspire to develop.

....
....
....
....
....
....
....
....
....
....
....
....
....

Consider the phrase "strength spotting." Look around, considering people on your team, your local barista, someone from the grocery store, or even a member of your family. Spot the strengths they demonstrate. One day, tell them how much you admire their strengths. How about today? Right now?

DAY 27: TAKE THE TEST

Character strengths define us as human beings, feeding our capacity to think, feel, act, and make decisions. Take the Character Strengths survey, a series of questions that are grounded in the work of the VIA (Values in Action) Institute. You'll need to create a free online account to do it, then you can wait for the results to hit your inbox. Here's the web address: www.viacharacter.org.

Which of your current projects align well with your strengths? Which are out of alignment? How do you know? What are you going to do about it? Options include: Accept. Reject. Change. Reframe.

Finally, are you happy with the results from the Character Strengths survey? If not, make a note to take the test again on another day.

DAY 28: ASK A FRIEND OR TWO

Make a copy of the list of 24 Character Strengths. Ask someone who knows you well to check off your top five strengths. Encourage them to choose quickly, without thinking too much. Do the same with someone who doesn't know you very well.

Asking for feedback makes us vulnerable. You now have at least three versions of your Character Strengths profile: your self-reflection, a computer-generated reflection, and the reflection of at least one other person. Compare various responses, knowing that feedback isn't necessarily true, false, or even accurate. It's just a reflection. What do you think? Do you accept them? Reject? Want to change? Reframe?

Two months from today: If you are eager to revisit this feedback, re-take the VIA test in two months. When you do, note how your various strengths move around.

DAY 29: PURE GRATITUDE

Make a list and be specific about the following: "My Five Favourite People, Places, Pets, or Things." Tell a story about something you are grateful for right here, right now.

....

....

....

....

....

....

....

....

....

....

....

....

When you intentionally practice gratitude and write daily, you'll start noting shifts in your health, relationships, and mood. Pay attention to the following:

- Sleep
- Appetite
- Energy levels
- Relationships at home, at work, and on teams
- Decisions related to time and resources
- Thought processes related to decision-making

DAY 30: WHO ARE YOU GOING TO THANK?

Think about someone you would like to thank. Make a plan to take this person on a friendly date. Perhaps the person you most want to thank is yourself. Grab a coffee, go for a rejuvenating bike ride, visit an art gallery, indulge at a spa. Do something special, and make joy and gratitude a part of your day. Pay attention, make notes, and seriously plan your outing.

Did you thank someone? How did it go? Did you set expectations ahead of time, or did you just roll with it? What did you learn? Where is your positive energy leading you next?

BONUS DAY: NOW TO KEEP GOING

Refer to Day 22, and consider your list of reasons you want to keep writing. Thirty days is an excellent beginning. If you want to make this writerly habit sustainable, you will need to keep writing and flexing your muscles for another 30 days, and then continue for another 30 days after that.

What challenges will you face in the coming weeks? How can your writing practice serve you? How can you set yourself up for success? Do you need an accountability buddy? Any other ideas? Add some notes to your writerly self.

....
....
....
....
....
....
....
....
....
....
....
....
....

APPENDIX

On Day 24, I invite you to look at the following list of Character Strengths, and check your top five strengths as a self-reflection.

On Day 26, I invite you to do some "strengths spotting" by noting the strengths of others, and putting names beside the strengths you spot in them.

On Day 27, I invite you to take the online survey at: www.viacharacter.org and note the top five strengths you receive.

On Day 28, I invite you to make a copy of this table and ask a close friend to put a check beside the five strengths they spot in you. Consider asking the same of someone who does not know you well.

The survey results are interpretations of your strengths rankings at a certain point in time. That said, change is a constant and life is dynamic. Consider re-taking the survey in a few months time.

VIA CLASSIFICATION OF CHARACTER STRENGTHS AND VIRTUES

© Copyright 2004-2023, VIA Institute on Character. All Rights Reserved. Used with Permission. www.viacharacter.org

Virtue of Wisdom: strengths that help you gather and use knowledge

- **Creativity:** Original and adaptive, shows ingenuity, sees and does things in different ways
- **Curiosity:** Interested, seeks novelty, appreciates exploration, open to experience
- **Judgment / Critical Thinking:** thinks through all sides, doesn't jump to conclusions
- **Love of Learning:** Interested in mastering new skills and information, systematically adds to knowledge
- **Perspective:** Wise, provides wise counsel, takes the big-picture view

Virtue of Courage: strengths that help you exercise your will and face adversity

- **Bravery:** Shows valor, doesn't shrink from threat or challenge, faces fears, speaks up for what's right
- **Perseverance:** Persistent, industrious, finishes what he or she starts, overcomes obstacles
- **Honesty:** Authentic, true to him or herself, sincere, shows integrity
- **Zest:** Vital, enthusiastic for life, vigorous, energetic, does things wholeheartedly

Virtue of Humanity: strengths that help you in one-on-one relationships

- **Love:** Both loving and loved, values close relations with others, shows genuine warmth
- **Kindness:** Generous, nurturing, caring, compassionate, altruistic, does for others
- **Social Intelligence:** Emotionally intelligent, aware of the motives and feelings of self and others, knows what makes other people tick

Virtue of Justice: strengths that help you in community or group-based situations

> **Teamwork:** A good citizen, socially responsible, loyal, contributes to group efforts
>
> **Fairness:** Adheres to principles of justice, doesn't let feelings bias decisions, offers equal opportunity to all
>
> **Leadership:** Organizes groups to get things done, positively guides others

Virtue of Temperance: strengths that help you manage habits and protect against excess

> **Forgiveness:** Merciful, accepting of others' shortcomings, gives people a second change, letting go of hurt when wronged
>
> **Humility:** Modest, lets his or her accomplishments speak for themselves
>
> **Prudence:** Careful about his or her choices, cautious, doesn't take undue risks
>
> **Self-Regulation:** Self-controlled, disciplined, able to manage impulses, emotions and vices

Virtue of Transcendence: strengths that help you connect to the larger universe and provide meaning

> **Appreciation of Beauty and Excellence:** Experiences awe and wonder for beauty, admires skills and excellence in others, elevated by moral beauty (goodness of others)
>
> **Gratitude:** Thankful for the good in life, expresses thanks, feels blessed
>
> **Hope:** Optimistic, positive and future minded, expects the best and works to achieve it
>
> **Humor:** Playful, brings smiles to others, lighthearted, sees the lighter side
>
> **Spirituality:** Having coherent beliefs about the higher purpose and meaning of the universe, knowing where one fits within the larger scheme, having beliefs about the meaning of life that shape conduct and provide comfort

POSTSCRIPT

During COVID-19, as I researched the science of gratitude, I grew to understand the remarkable benefits of writing longhand, a habit I have been practicing for almost 30 years. As I read about the significance of building habits of mind, habits remembered, and habits shaped by our lived experiences, my Grassroots Gratitude brainchild was growing.

My book, *An Ecology of Gratitude: Writing Your Way to What Matters*, went live in November 2021. It has become the solid launching pad and the vision behind my social purpose venture, Grassroots Gratitude, and fuel for this *Gratitude Ignition Guide*.

Grassroots Gratitude is a legacy project, and I am motivated by the following mission: To foster gratitude as the secret strength of everyday leadership, every day.

By fostering gratitude, Grassroots Gratitude hopes to ignite positivity and possibility in the imaginations of all who hold leadership roles. Join me in imagining a brighter future for the next generation, and generations beyond, so we can create and enjoy a world where we thrive in an environment of clean air, clean water, healthy soils, and right-fitting relationships for decades to come.

How will you stoke your gratitude fires and keep writing your way to what matters in the days, months, and years to come? By finding your reasons to be grateful, your motivation to live each day with purpose will intensify. Keep going with gratitude. Keep writing in your journal. Remember to savour the good stuff. Align your efforts by networking with good

Postscript

people doing good things and stay connected to Grassroots Gratitude. How?

- Find an accountability buddy.
- Sign up for a workshop: grassrootsgratitude.ca/programs-and-events/.
- Purchase copies of my book(s) as gifts for your organization or colleagues. Bulk discounts are available grassrootsgratitude.ca/your-personal-gratitude-guide/.
- Subscribe to my grateful blog at www.grassrootsgratitude.ca.
- Subscribe to my YouTube channel: @grassrootsgratitude.
- Attend events (virtual and in person).
- Take advantage of free resources found on my website and invite a friend to do the same.
- Connect with me. Together, let's imagine a grateful project, either for you as an individual, or as part of a leadership group.
- Invite me to your next learning and development session, virtual or face-to-face.
- Contact me: lorraine@grassrootsgratitude.ca. I love hearing about any bold, audacious, and grateful goals, and am always eager to learn how this *Gratitude Ignition Guide* has impacted your leadership self.

Time for you to take the tiller and notice the shifts in your life and patterns of thinking. Ready to shift and then shift some more? Let me know if I can help you with your next writing shift.

Lorraine Widmer-Carson

CITATIONS

1. Kaufman, S. B. (2015, August 2). "Which Character Strengths Are Most Predictive of Well-Being?." Scientific American Blog Network. https://blogs.scientificamerican.com/beautiful-minds/which-character-strengths-are-most-predictive-of-well-being/.
2. Summer, A. "The Science of Gratitude." (2018, May). A white paper prepared for the John Templeton Foundation by the Greater Good Science Center at UC Berkeley. https://ggsc.berkeley.edu/images/uploads/GGSC-JTF_White_Paper-Gratitude-FINAL.pdf.
3. Hanson, R. (2018, November 29). "Gratitude and the 'Buddha Brain.'" Dr. Rick Hanson. https://www.rickhanson.net/gratitude-buddha-brain/.
4. Marsh, J. (2011, November 17). "Tips for Keeping a Gratitude Journal." Greater Good. https://greatergood.berkeley.edu/article/item/tips_for_keeping_a_gratitude_journal.
5. Buffo, J. (@022, March 21) "Untangling You: How Can I Be Grateful When I Feel So Resentful." WellRx https://www.wellrx.com/news/how-a-gratitude-journal-can-support-your-mental-health/.
6. Emmons, Robert A. *Thanks! How Practicing Gratitude Can Make You Happier.* Houghton Mifflin Harcourt Publishing Company. 2007.
7. Keltner, D. K. U. B. D., & Jason Marsh (n.d.). "How Gratitude Beats Materialism." Greater Good. https://greatergood.berkeley.edu/article/item/materialism_gratitude_happiness.
8. Staff, Insperity. (2023, July 11). Insperity. "5 Essential Traits of Effective Everyday Leadership." https://www.insperity.com/blog/everyday-leadership/.
9. Simard, Suzanne: *Finding the Mother Tree: Discovering the Wisdom of the Forest.* Penguin Canada, a division of Penguin Random House Canada Limited. 2021.
10. Seligman, Martin E.P. *Authentic Happiness: Using New Positive Psychology to Realize Your Potential for Lasting Fulfillment.* The Free Press, A Division of Simon and Schuster, Inc. 2002.
11. Waldinger, Robert and Marc Schulz. *The Good Life: Lessons from the World's Longest Scientific Study of Happiness.* Simon & Shuster. 2023.
12. Fredrickson, Barbara L. *Positivity: Discover the Upward Spiral That Will Change Your Life.* Harmony Books. 2009.

Citations

13. Courtney E. Ackerman, MA. (2023, September 18). "15 Character Strength Examples, Interventions & Worksheets." PositivePsychology.com. https://positivepsychology.com/character-strength-examples-interventions-worksheets/.
14. Schwartz, Richard C. No Bad Parts: *Healing Trauma and Restoring Wellness with the Internal Family Systems Model*. Sounds True. 2021.
15. Niemiec, Ryan M. and Robert E. McGrath. *The Power of Character Strengths: Appreciate and Ignite Your Positive Personality*. An Official Guide from the VIA Institute on Character. 2019.

MORE READING RESOURCES FOR EVERYDAY LEADERS

Block, Peter. *Community: The Structure of Belonging.* Berrett-Koehler Publishers, Inc. 2009.

Brown, Brené. *The Gifts of Imperfection: Let Go of Who You Think You're Supposed to Be and Embrace Who You Are.* Hazelden Publishing. 2010.

Brown, Brené. *Atlas of the Heart: Mapping Meaningful Connection and the Language of the Human Experience.* Random House. 2021.

Emmons, Robert A. *Gratitude Works! A 21-Day Program for Creating Emotional Prosperity.* Jossey-Bass. 2013.

Emmons, Robert A. *The Little Book of Gratitude: Create a Life of Happiness and Wellbeing by Giving Thanks.* Octopus Publishing Group Ltd. 2016.

Howells, Kerry. *Untangling You. How can I be grateful when I feel so resentful?* Major Street Publishing Pty Ltd. 2021.

Lyubomirsky, Sonja. *A New Approach to Getting the Life You Want.* Penguin Books. 2007.

Pipher, Mary. *Writing to Change the World.* The Berkley Publishing Group, Published by the Penguin Group. 2006.

Seligman, Martin E.P. Flourish: *Visionary New Understanding of Happiness and Well-being.* Atria Paperback. A Division of Simon & Shuster, Inc. 2011.

ABOUT THE AUTHOR

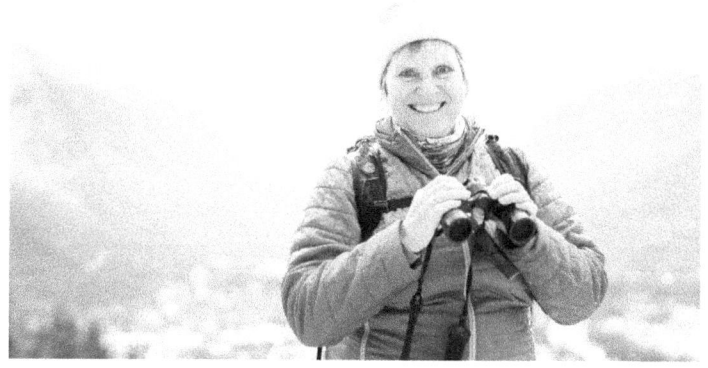

With more than 10,000 hours of practice across 150 journals, Lorraine Widmer-Carson's daily habit of thoughtful and introspective writing continues to ground her work as a socially conscious and active community change maker. Today, she serves in a variety of educational and communications roles, and applies the everyday leadership lessons she learned as a mother of four, a business owner, a ski-racing mama and the founding executive director of The Banff Canmore Community Foundation. Her first book, *An Ecology of Gratitude: Writing Your Way to What Matters,* was released in November 2021. In this second publication, *Gratitude Ignition Guide: Notes for My Leadership Self,* she seeks to support everyday leaders who want to hone their positivity and communication skills in order to lead with greater self awareness, self acceptance, and humility.

www.ingramcontent.com/pod-product-compliance
Lightning Source LLC
Chambersburg PA
CBHW060033040426
42333CB00042B/2418